Dummies type 2 diabetes guide 2024

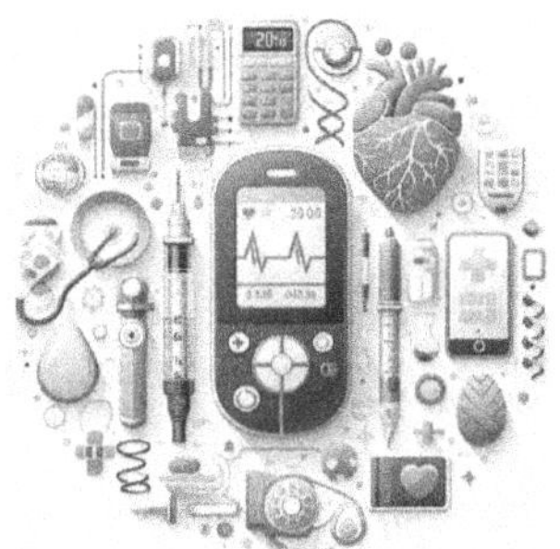

The Ultimate Guide to Living a Healthy Life and Managing a Newly Diagnosed Type 2 Diabetes with a 30-Day Meal Plan and Easy, Sample Low-carb Recipes.

Dr. Stephen Campbell

Table of Contents

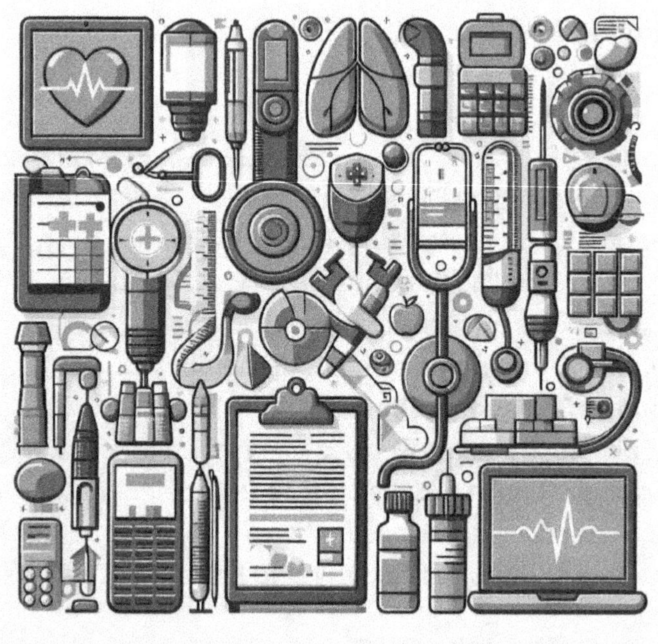

Introduction

The past three years had been difficult for Lisa, a 42-year-old woman who had type 2 diabetes. She had experimented with a number of drugs and lifestyle modifications in an effort to manage her blood sugar, but nothing appeared to be working. She was starting to feel dejected and frustrated.

A book titled "Dummies type 2 diabetes guide" was discovered by Lisa one day while she was perusing a nearby bookstore. She chose to read it because she found the title intriguing.

The value of a healthy diet and regular exercise in controlling type 2 diabetes was covered in the book. The many accessible pharmaceutical types were also described, along with any possible side effects. The information captivated Lisa, who made the decision to test it out.

She began by altering her dietary habits and consuming more nutritious grains, fruits, and veggies. She started going to the gym frequently and making sure she got plenty of rest. After a few weeks, Lisa discovered to her joyful surprise that her blood sugar levels were improving.

Lisa proceeded to alter her way of life and food during the ensuing few months. Eventually, she succeeded in reversing her type 2 diabetes. She couldn't believe she could do this without taking any medication, and she was relieved.

What is Diabetes?

Diabetes is a chronic metabolic disorder characterized by elevated levels of glucose in the blood. Glucose, a type of sugar, serves as the body's primary source of energy and is derived from the food we eat. Insulin, a hormone produced by the pancreas, plays a crucial role in regulating glucose levels by facilitating its uptake into cells.

In individuals with diabetes, either the body does not produce enough insulin (insulin deficiency) or the cells become resistant to the effects of insulin (insulin resistance), leading to impaired glucose metabolism. This results in elevated blood sugar levels, a condition known as hyperglycemia, which can have detrimental effects on various organs and systems in the body if left untreated.

Different Types of Diabetes

There are several types of diabetes, each with its own distinct etiology, characteristics, and management strategies. The most common types include:

- **Type 1 Diabetes**: This form of diabetes is characterized by autoimmune destruction of the insulin-producing beta cells in the pancreas, leading to absolute insulin deficiency. Type 1 diabetes typically develops during childhood or adolescence and requires lifelong insulin therapy for management.

- **Type 2 Diabetes**: Type 2 diabetes accounts for the majority of diabetes cases and is characterized by insulin resistance and relative insulin deficiency. It is often associated with lifestyle factors such as obesity, sedentary behavior, and unhealthy dietary habits, although genetic predisposition also plays a role. Type 2 diabetes can often be managed through lifestyle modifications, oral medications, and insulin therapy if needed.

- **Gestational Diabetes**: Gestational diabetes occurs during pregnancy and is characterized by elevated blood sugar levels that develop or are first recognized during pregnancy. While gestational diabetes usually resolves after childbirth, it increases the risk of complications for both the mother and baby and may predispose the mother to developing type 2 diabetes later in life.

How it is Diagnosed

Diabetes is diagnosed through various blood tests that measure blood glucose levels. The most common tests include:

- Fasting Plasma Glucose Test: This test measures blood glucose levels after fasting for at least eight hours. A fasting blood glucose level of 126 milligrams per deciliter (mg/dL) or higher on two separate occasions indicates diabetes.

- Oral Glucose Tolerance Test (OGTT): This test involves drinking a sugary solution, followed by blood glucose measurements at specified intervals. A blood glucose level of 200 mg/dL or higher two hours after consuming the glucose solution indicates diabetes.

- Hemoglobin A1c Test: This test measures the average blood glucose levels over the past two to three months. An A1c level of 6.5% or higher indicates diabetes.

Understanding Diabetes

Understanding diabetes involves knowing how the body normally processes glucose and how this process is disrupted in individuals with diabetes. It also entails recognizing the risk factors, symptoms, and potential complications associated with the condition. By understanding diabetes, individuals can make informed decisions about their health and take proactive steps to manage the condition effectively.

Who Else has Diabetes

Diabetes affects people of all ages, races, and backgrounds worldwide. While certain populations may have a higher prevalence of diabetes due to genetic predisposition, lifestyle factors, socioeconomic status, or access to healthcare, the condition can affect anyone. Family history, obesity, physical inactivity, poor dietary habits, and aging are common risk factors for diabetes, but environmental factors and individual behaviors also play significant roles in disease development. Therefore, raising awareness about diabetes and promoting preventive measures are crucial for addressing this growing public health concern.

Chapter 1:Understanding Type 2 Diabetes

Type 2 diabetes is a complex metabolic disorder characterized by high blood sugar levels, insulin resistance, and relative insulin deficiency. To comprehend the intricacies of this condition, it's essential to delve into the mechanisms of glucose metabolism and the role of insulin in the body.

At its core, type 2 diabetes arises when the body becomes resistant to the effects of insulin, a hormone produced by the pancreas. Insulin plays a crucial role in regulating blood sugar levels by facilitating the uptake of glucose into cells, where it can be used for energy production. However, in individuals with insulin resistance, cells become less responsive to insulin's signals, leading to impaired glucose uptake and elevated blood sugar levels.

Various factors contribute to the development of insulin resistance, including genetics, obesity, sedentary lifestyle, and dietary habits. Genetic predisposition can increase the likelihood of developing insulin resistance, while excess body weight, particularly abdominal fat, exacerbates the condition. Furthermore, a sedentary lifestyle and poor dietary choices, such as consuming high-calorie, processed foods, can further impair insulin sensitivity.

As insulin resistance progresses, the pancreas compensates by producing more insulin to maintain normal blood sugar levels. However, over time, the pancreas may fail to keep up with the increased demand for insulin production, leading to relative insulin deficiency. This imbalance between insulin resistance and insulin secretion ultimately results in elevated blood sugar levels characteristic of type 2 diabetes.

In addition to insulin resistance and relative insulin deficiency, other metabolic abnormalities contribute to the pathophysiology of type 2 diabetes. These may include dysfunction of pancreatic alpha and beta cells, impaired incretin hormone signaling, increased hepatic glucose production, and altered adipokine secretion from adipose tissue.

Understanding the underlying mechanisms of type 2 diabetes is crucial for effective management and treatment. By addressing insulin resistance, promoting healthy lifestyle habits, and optimizing glucose metabolism, individuals with type 2 diabetes can better control their blood sugar levels and reduce the risk of complications associated with the condition.

Understanding the Causes of Type 2 Diabetes

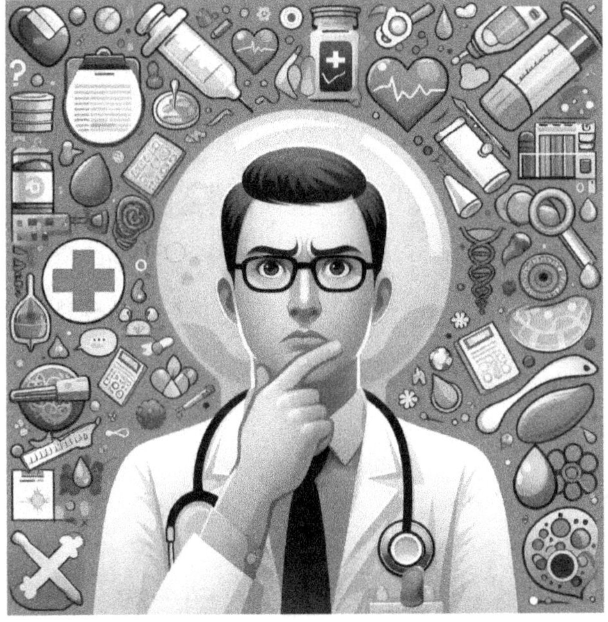

Millions of individuals worldwide suffer with type 2 diabetes, a chronic disease that is brought on by a combination of environmental, genetic, and lifestyle factors. High blood sugar levels are a defining feature of the illness, which can cause a number of major health issues.

You can lower your risk of getting type 2 diabetes by taking action by being aware of its causes.

Genetics

Diabetes type 2 is influenced by genetics. You might be more prone to developing the ailment if it runs in your family. According to research, people of particular races and ethnicities are more likely to develop type 2 diabetes.

Age

Your risk of type 2 diabetes may also be impacted by your age. Your risk increases as you age. Type 2 diabetes is more likely to strike adults over the age of 45 than it is younger ones.

Weight

Obesity and being overweight are significant risk factors for type 2 diabetes. The body's capacity to react to insulin, the hormone that aids in controlling blood sugar levels, can be lowered by obesity. Type 2 diabetes is more likely to strike overweight people than healthy-weight people.

Diet

You run a higher risk of developing type 2 diabetes if you consume a diet heavy in refined carbs, such as white bread and sugary beverages. Consuming excessive amounts of fried and processed food can also raise your risk.

Physical exercise

Another risk factor for type 2 diabetes is physical inactivity. Inactivity increases the likelihood of developing the illness compared to regular exercise.

Lifestyle

Your risk of type 2 diabetes may also rise if you smoke, consume alcohol, or sleep insufficiently. Stressed-out individuals may also be more prone to developing the illness.

You can lower your risk of getting type 2 diabetes by taking action after learning the causes of the disease. Your risk can be decreased by making lifestyle changes like eating a healthy diet, exercising frequently, and giving up smoking. A frequent health checkup might help you keep track of your risk of type 2 diabetes.

Diagnosis and Initial Steps

In the journey of life, there are moments that test our courage and resilience, moments that beckon us to confront the unknown with steadfast determination. For those who find themselves at the crossroads of diabetes diagnosis, such moments can be fraught with uncertainty and fear. Yet, amid the shadows of doubt, there shines a beacon of hope – the promise of diagnosis and the initial steps toward reclaiming control of one's health.

The journey begins with awareness – a gentle whisper that stirs the soul and prompts us to listen to the whispers of our bodies. Symptoms such as increased thirst, frequent urination, unexplained weight loss, and fatigue serve as harbingers of change, urging us to heed the call of self-care and seek answers to the questions that linger in the recesses of our minds.

But it is not until we stand face to face with the truth – the reality of a diabetes diagnosis – that the weight of our journey truly begins to bear down upon us. In that moment of revelation, emotions may run high, ranging from disbelief and denial to anger and despair. It is natural to feel overwhelmed by the enormity of the task that lies ahead, but remember, you are not alone.

With diagnosis comes clarity – a newfound understanding of the path that lies before us and the steps we must take to navigate its twists and turns. The journey begins with acceptance – a gentle surrender to the truth of our condition and a commitment to take charge of our health with courage and resolve.

The initial steps may seem daunting, but they are the foundation upon which our journey toward wellness is built. It begins with education – arming ourselves with knowledge and empowering ourselves with the tools we need to manage our diabetes effectively. Through guidance from healthcare professionals, we learn to monitor our blood sugar levels, understand the importance of medication adherence, and embrace lifestyle modifications that promote optimal health.

But the journey is not without its challenges. Along the way, we may encounter obstacles that test our resolve and shake our confidence. It is in these moments of struggle that we must summon our inner strength and lean on the support of others. Whether through the encouragement of loved ones, the wisdom of healthcare providers, or the camaraderie of support groups, we find solace in knowing that we are not alone on this path.

As we take our first tentative steps forward, let us do so with hope in our hearts and determination in our souls. For though the road ahead may be long and arduous, it is also filled with promise and possibility. With each passing day, we grow stronger, more resilient, and more capable of overcoming the challenges that lie in our path.

In the chapters that follow, we will delve deeper into the intricacies of diabetes management, exploring the strategies and techniques that will empower us to take control of our health and live our lives to the fullest. Let us embark on this journey together, united in our commitment to wellness and inspired by the strength that lies within us all.

Chapter 2 : managing type 2 diabetes

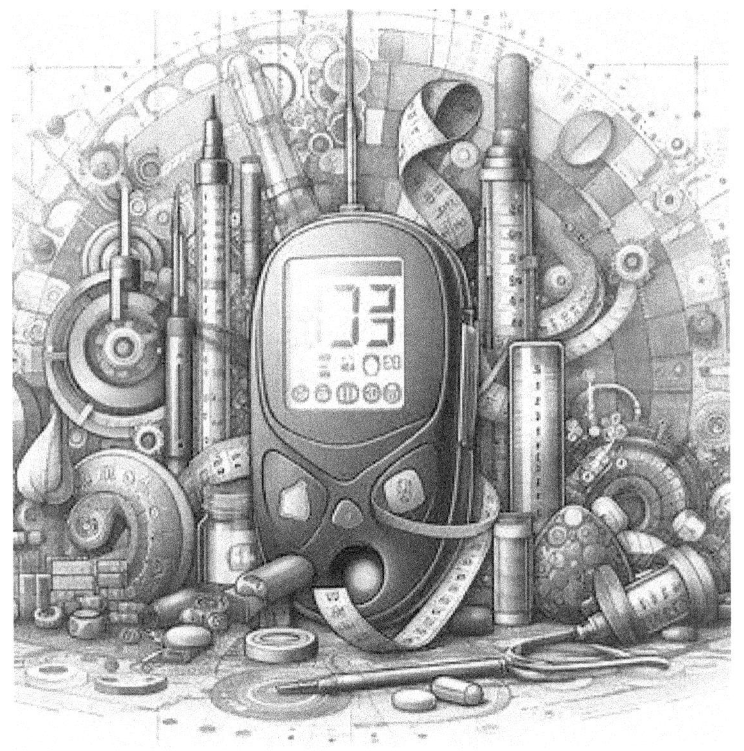

Following are some guidelines for controlling type 2 diabetes:

1. Regularly check your blood glucose levels. Doing this will enable you to see any changes in your levels and take the necessary action. A blood glucose meter can be used for this, or your doctor can check your levels on a regular basis.

2. Consume a nutritious diet: Maintaining a healthy diet is crucial for controlling type 2 diabetes. A balanced diet high in fiber, fruits, vegetables, and whole grains, low in sugar and saturated fat, and low in saturated fat and sugar can help you maintain stable blood sugar levels and avoid issues.

3. frequent exercise: Keeping your type 2 diabetes under control requires frequent exercise. Your body's sensitivity to insulin can be improved and blood glucose levels can be lowered with regular exercise. On most days of the week, try to get in at least 30 minutes of moderate exercise, such as walking, cycling, or swimming.

4. Take meds as directed: It's vital to follow your doctor's instructions if you've been given medication to manage type 2 diabetes. This can help you maintain appropriate blood sugar levels and avoid any problems.

5. Control your stress levels: Stress can increase blood sugar levels, therefore it's critical to control it to keep them within a healthy range. Exercises for reducing stress, such yoga, meditation, and mindfulness, can be beneficial.

6. Keep an eye on your feet: Diabetics are more prone to foot issues including infections and ulcers. Regularly inspect your feet for any injury or infection symptoms, and get medical help if necessary.

7. Give up smoking: If you smoke, it's vital to stop because it might make type 2 diabetes symptoms worse. You can stop smoking with the aid of numerous tools, including counseling and nicotine replacement therapy.

8. Embrace the Healing Power of Nature: Amidst the hustle and bustle of modern life, find solace in the tranquility of nature's embrace. Take time each day to connect with the world around you – whether through a leisurely stroll in the park, a hike through the forest, or a moment of quiet reflection by the water's edge. In the serenity of nature's embrace, find respite from the stresses of daily life and nourish your soul with the healing power of the natural world.

9. Cultivate Joyful Moments: In the midst of life's challenges, seek out moments of joy and laughter to uplift your spirits and lighten your heart. Whether it's sharing a laugh with loved ones, indulging in a favorite hobby, or simply savoring the small pleasures of everyday life, find moments of joy that ignite your soul and fill your heart with warmth. In the presence of joy, find strength to face the challenges of managing type 2 diabetes with grace and resilience.

10. Foster Connection and Community: Reach out to others who share your journey and find strength in the bonds of community and connection. Whether

it's joining a support group, participating in online forums, or connecting with others through social media, surround yourself with a network of support and encouragement. In the company of kindred spirits, find solace in shared experiences and discover the power of collective resilience in overcoming the challenges of type 2 diabetes.

11. Practice Gratitude and Mindfulness: Cultivate a spirit of gratitude and mindfulness to find peace and contentment amidst life's challenges. Take time each day to reflect on the blessings in your life – whether it's the love of family and friends, the beauty of nature, or the simple joys of everyday living. In the practice of gratitude, find strength to face the ups and downs of managing type 2 diabetes with grace and acceptance.

12. Seek Professional Support: Reach out to healthcare professionals who can provide guidance and support in managing type 2 diabetes. Whether it's working with a registered dietitian to develop a personalized meal plan, consulting with an exercise physiologist to design an exercise program tailored to your needs, or seeking the expertise of a mental health

professional to address stress and emotional well-being, surround yourself with a team of experts who can help you navigate the complexities of type 2 diabetes with confidence and compassion

Chapter 3:Diabetes Diet and Nutrition

In the journey of managing diabetes, the food we eat becomes not just nourishment, but a powerful tool for maintaining our health and well-being. Like pieces of a puzzle, each meal plays a crucial role in keeping our blood sugar levels stable and our bodies thriving.

1. **Low-Carb Diet**: Picture a plate filled with lean proteins like chicken, fish, and tofu, alongside healthy fats from avocados, nuts, and olive oil. By reducing the intake of carbohydrates found in bread, pasta, and sugary snacks, a low-carb diet helps to stabilize blood sugar levels and promote weight loss. With each bite, we nourish our bodies with the building blocks of health, paving the way for a brighter, healthier future.

2. **Mediterranean Diet**: Transport yourself to the sun-drenched shores of the Mediterranean, where the air is filled with the scent of fresh herbs and the promise of wholesome, flavorful cuisine. Embracing

the Mediterranean diet means savoring the vibrant colors and flavors of fruits, vegetables, whole grains, and heart-healthy fats like olive oil and nuts. With each meal, we indulge in a symphony of tastes and textures, nourishing not just our bodies, but our souls.

3. **High Fiber Diet**: Imagine a garden bursting with life – rows of leafy greens, plump tomatoes, and colorful bell peppers stretching toward the sky. This is the essence of a high-fiber diet, rich in whole grains, legumes, fruits, and vegetables. With each bite, we fuel our bodies with the roughage and nutrients they crave, supporting digestion, stabilizing blood sugar levels, and promoting a sense of fullness and satisfaction.

4. **Low Glycemic Index Diet**: Envision a table set with foods that release their energy slowly, like a gentle stream flowing through the countryside. This is the essence of a low glycemic index diet, which focuses on consuming foods that are digested and absorbed gradually, helping to keep blood sugar levels steady throughout the day. By choosing foods like non-starchy vegetables, whole grains, and

legumes, we create a foundation of stability and balance in our diets.

5. **Ketogenic Diet:** Journey into the realm of the ketogenic diet, where fats reign supreme and carbs are kept to a minimum. In this eating plan, the body enters a state of ketosis, burning fat for fuel instead of glucose. While traditionally used for weight loss, research suggests that a ketogenic diet may also benefit those with type 2 diabetes by improving insulin sensitivity and blood sugar control. With each meal, we embrace the power of fat as fuel, unlocking a new realm of possibility for managing our diabetes.

Remember, there is no one-size-fits-all approach to diabetic diet and nutrition. Each person is unique, with their own individual needs and preferences. By working with a licensed dietitian, we can tailor our eating plans to meet our specific requirements, ensuring that we receive the nutrition we need to thrive. In the journey of managing diabetes, food becomes not just sustenance, but a source of empowerment, helping us to take control of our health and live our lives to the fullest.

Simple Breakfast Recipes for type 2 diabetes

Breakfast Recipe 1: Veggie Omelette

Introduction:

Start your day off right with this delicious and nutritious veggie omelette, perfect for managing type 2 diabetes. Packed with protein and fiber, this hearty breakfast will keep you feeling satisfied and energized throughout the morning.

Carb Counting: Approximately 10 grams of carbohydrates per serving.

Nutritional Information:
- Calories: 250
- Total Fat: 15g
- Saturated Fat: 5g
- Cholesterol: 280mg
- Sodium: 450mg
- Total Carbohydrates: 10g
- Dietary Fiber: 3g
- Sugars: 2g

- Protein: 20g

Serving Size: 1 omelette

Prep Time: 10 minutes

Ingredients:
- 2 large eggs
- 1/4 cup diced bell peppers
- 1/4 cup diced onions
- 1/4 cup diced tomatoes
- 1/4 cup chopped spinach
- 1/4 cup shredded low-fat cheese
- Salt and pepper to taste
- Cooking spray

Instructions:
1. In a small bowl, beat the eggs with a fork until well combined. Season with salt and pepper to taste.
2. Heat a non-stick skillet over medium heat and lightly coat with cooking spray.
3. Add the diced bell peppers, onions, and tomatoes to the skillet and sauté until softened, about 2-3 minutes.

4. Add the chopped spinach to the skillet and cook until wilted, about 1 minute.

5. Pour the beaten eggs over the cooked vegetables in the skillet, tilting the pan to evenly distribute the eggs.

6. Cook the omelette for 2-3 minutes, or until the edges begin to set.

7. Sprinkle the shredded cheese evenly over one half of the omelette.

8. Using a spatula, carefully fold the other half of the omelette over the cheese to form a half-moon shape.

9. Cook for an additional 1-2 minutes, or until the cheese is melted and the eggs are fully cooked through.

10. Slide the omelette onto a plate and serve hot.

Enjoy your veggie omelette with a side of whole grain toast or fresh fruit for a balanced and satisfying breakfast.

(Note: Carb counting and nutritional information are approximate and may vary depending on specific ingredients and portion sizes used.)

Breakfast Recipe 2: Greek Yogurt Parfait

Introduction:

Indulge in a delightful Greek yogurt parfait that's not only delicious but also diabetes-friendly. This refreshing breakfast option is rich in protein and low in carbohydrates, making it an ideal choice for starting your day on the right foot.

Carb Counting: Approximately 15 grams of carbohydrates per serving.

Nutritional Information:

- Calories: 200
- Total Fat: 5g
- Saturated Fat: 2g
- Cholesterol: 10mg
- Sodium: 80mg
- Total Carbohydrates: 15g
- Dietary Fiber: 2g
- Sugars: 10g
- Protein: 15g

Serving Size: 1 parfait

Prep Time: 5 minutes

Ingredients:

- 1/2 cup plain Greek yogurt
- 1/4 cup fresh berries (such as strawberries, blueberries, or raspberries)
- 1 tablespoon chopped nuts (such as almonds or walnuts)
- 1 teaspoon honey or low-sugar fruit preserves
- 1 tablespoon granola (optional)
- Cinnamon for garnish (optional)

Instructions:

1. In a serving glass or bowl, layer the plain Greek yogurt at the bottom.
2. Add a layer of fresh berries on top of the yogurt.
3. Sprinkle the chopped nuts over the berries.
4. Drizzle the honey or spread the fruit preserves evenly over the nuts.
5. Repeat the layering process with the remaining yogurt, berries, nuts, and honey or fruit preserves.
6. If desired, sprinkle granola over the top for added crunch and texture.
7. Garnish with a dash of cinnamon for extra flavor.
8. Serve immediately and enjoy your delightful Greek yogurt parfait!

This satisfying breakfast option is not only delicious but also provides a balanced combination of protein, healthy fats, and carbohydrates to keep you feeling full and energized throughout the morning.

(Note: Carb counting and nutritional information are approximate and may vary depending on specific ingredients and portion sizes used.)

Breakfast Recipe 3: Avocado Toast

Introduction:

Savor the simplicity and nourishment of avocado toast, a beloved breakfast classic that's perfect for managing type 2 diabetes. With its combination of healthy fats, fiber, and protein, this quick and easy meal will keep you satisfied and fueled for the day ahead.

Carb Counting: Approximately 20 grams of carbohydrates per serving.

Nutritional Information:
- Calories: 300
- Total Fat: 15g

- Saturated Fat: 2g
- Cholesterol: 0mg
- Sodium: 200mg
- Total Carbohydrates: 20g
- Dietary Fiber: 7g
- Sugars: 2g
- Protein: 8g

Serving Size: 1 slice of toast

Prep Time: 5 minutes

Ingredients:

- 1 slice whole grain bread
- 1/2 ripe avocado
- 1 teaspoon lemon juice
- Salt and pepper to taste
- Optional toppings: sliced tomato, poached egg, microgreens, hot sauce

Instructions:

1. Toast the slice of whole grain bread until golden brown and crispy.
2. While the bread is toasting, scoop the flesh of the ripe avocado into a small bowl.

3. Add the lemon juice, salt, and pepper to the avocado, and mash with a fork until smooth and creamy.
4. Once the toast is done, spread the mashed avocado evenly over the surface.
5. Top with your desired toppings, such as sliced tomato, a poached egg, or a sprinkle of microgreens.
6. Season with additional salt and pepper to taste, if desired.
7. Serve immediately and enjoy your delicious and nutritious avocado toast!

This simple yet satisfying breakfast option is packed with heart-healthy fats, fiber, and nutrients to fuel your body and support your overall health and well-being.

(Note: Carb counting and nutritional information are approximate and may vary depending on specific ingredients and portion sizes used.)

Simple Lunch recipes for type 2 diabetes

Lunch Recipe 1: Grilled Chicken Salad

Introduction:

Savor the vibrant flavors and wholesome goodness of a grilled chicken salad, a perfect choice for managing type 2 diabetes. Bursting with fresh ingredients and protein-packed chicken, this salad will leave you feeling satisfied and energized to tackle the rest of your day.

Carb Counting: Approximately 15 grams of carbohydrates per serving.

Nutritional Information:
- Calories: 300
- Total Fat: 12g
- Saturated Fat: 2g
- Cholesterol: 80mg
- Sodium: 350mg
- Total Carbohydrates: 15g
- Dietary Fiber: 5g
- Sugars: 5g
- Protein: 25g

Serving Size: 1 salad

Prep Time: 15 minutes

Ingredients:

- 2 cups mixed salad greens (such as spinach, arugula, and romaine)
- 4 oz grilled chicken breast, sliced
- 1/4 cup cherry tomatoes, halved
- 1/4 cup cucumber, sliced
- 1/4 cup bell peppers, diced
- 1/4 cup carrots, shredded
- 2 tablespoons balsamic vinaigrette dressing
- Salt and pepper to taste
- Optional toppings: avocado slices, feta cheese, toasted nuts

Instructions:

1. In a large bowl, toss together the mixed salad greens, cherry tomatoes, cucumber, bell peppers, and carrots.
2. Top the salad with the sliced grilled chicken breast.
3. Drizzle the balsamic vinaigrette dressing over the salad and toss to coat evenly.

4. Season with salt and pepper to taste.

5. Divide the salad onto plates and garnish with optional toppings such as avocado slices, crumbled feta cheese, or toasted nuts.

6. Serve immediately and enjoy your delicious and nutritious grilled chicken salad!

This satisfying lunch option provides a balanced combination of protein, fiber, and essential nutrients to keep you feeling full and satisfied until dinner.

(Note: Carb counting and nutritional information are approximate and may vary depending on specific ingredients and portion sizes used.)

Lunch Recipe 2: Quinoa and Vegetable Stir-Fry

<u>Introduction:</u>

Transport your taste buds to the Far East with a flavorful quinoa and vegetable stir-fry, a diabetes-friendly lunch option that's as delicious as it is nutritious. Packed with protein-rich quinoa and an assortment of colorful vegetables, this stir-fry will tantalize your senses and nourish your body from the inside out.

Carb Counting: Approximately 30 grams of carbohydrates per serving.

Nutritional Information:

- Calories: 350
- Total Fat: 10g
- Saturated Fat: 1g
- Cholesterol: 0mg
- Sodium: 450mg
- Total Carbohydrates: 30g
- Dietary Fiber: 6g
- Sugars: 5g
- Protein: 15g

Serving Size: 1 bowl

Prep Time: 20 minutes

Ingredients:

- 1/2 cup quinoa, rinsed and drained
- 1 cup water or low-sodium vegetable broth
- 1 tablespoon olive oil
- 2 cloves garlic, minced
- 1 cup mixed vegetables (such as bell peppers, broccoli, snap peas, and carrots)

- 2 tablespoons low-sodium soy sauce
- 1 tablespoon rice vinegar
- 1 teaspoon sesame oil
- Salt and pepper to taste
- Optional toppings: sliced green onions, toasted sesame seeds

Instructions:

1. In a small saucepan, bring the water or vegetable broth to a boil. Add the quinoa, reduce the heat to low, cover, and simmer for 15 minutes, or until the quinoa is cooked and the liquid is absorbed.
2. While the quinoa is cooking, heat the olive oil in a large skillet or wok over medium-high heat. Add the minced garlic and cook for 1 minute, or until fragrant.
3. Add the mixed vegetables to the skillet and stir-fry for 3-4 minutes, or until crisp-tender.
4. In a small bowl, whisk together the soy sauce, rice vinegar, and sesame oil.
5. Add the cooked quinoa to the skillet with the vegetables and pour the soy sauce mixture over the top. Stir to combine and heat through.
6. Season with salt and pepper to taste.

7. Divide the quinoa and vegetable stir-fry into bowls and garnish with optional toppings such as sliced green onions or toasted sesame seeds.

8. Serve immediately and enjoy your flavorful and nutritious quinoa and vegetable stir-fry!

This satisfying lunch option is not only delicious but also provides a balanced combination of protein, fiber, and essential nutrients to keep you feeling full and satisfied until dinner.

(Note: Carb counting and nutritional information are approximate and may vary depending on specific ingredients and portion sizes used.)

Lunch Recipe 3: Turkey and Avocado Wrap

<u>Introduction:</u>

Treat yourself to a tasty and satisfying turkey and avocado wrap, perfect for managing type 2 diabetes. Packed with lean protein, healthy fats, and plenty of fresh veggies, this wrap is a delicious and nutritious option for lunchtime.

Carb Counting: Approximately 25 grams of carbohydrates per serving.

Nutritional Information:

- Calories: 320
- Total Fat: 15g
- Saturated Fat: 2g
- Cholesterol: 30mg
- Sodium: 400mg
- Total Carbohydrates: 25g
- Dietary Fiber: 5g
- Sugars: 3g
- Protein: 20g

Serving Size: 1 wrap

Prep Time: 10 minutes

Ingredients:

- 1 whole grain tortilla or wrap
- 3 oz sliced turkey breast
- 1/4 ripe avocado, mashed
- 1/4 cup shredded lettuce or baby spinach
- 2 slices tomato
- 2 slices cucumber
- 1 tablespoon hummus or mustard
- Salt and pepper to taste

<u>**Instructions:**</u>

1. Lay the whole grain tortilla or wrap flat on a clean surface.
2. Spread the mashed avocado evenly over the surface of the tortilla.
3. Layer the sliced turkey breast, shredded lettuce or baby spinach, tomato slices, and cucumber slices on top of the avocado.
4. Spread the hummus or mustard over the filling.
5. Season with salt and pepper to taste.
6. Roll up the tortilla tightly, folding in the sides as you go.
7. Slice the wrap in half diagonally and serve immediately.

Enjoy your delicious and nutritious turkey and avocado wrap with a side of fresh fruit or a small salad for a balanced and satisfying lunch.

(Note: Carb counting and nutritional information are approximate and may vary depending on specific ingredients and portion sizes used.)

Simple Dinner recipes for types 2 diabetes

Dinner Recipe 1: Baked Salmon with Roasted Vegetables

Introduction:

End your day on a high note with this delightful dinner of baked salmon and roasted vegetables, perfect for managing type 2 diabetes. Bursting with flavor and packed with nutrients, this wholesome meal will leave you feeling satisfied and nourished from the inside out.

Carb Counting: Approximately 20 grams of carbohydrates per serving.

Nutritional Information:

- Calories: 350
- Total Fat: 15g
- Saturated Fat: 2g
- Cholesterol: 80mg
- Sodium: 400mg
- Total Carbohydrates: 20g

- Dietary Fiber: 6g
- Sugars: 8g
- Protein: 25g

Serving Size: 1 fillet of salmon with vegetables

Prep Time: 20 minutes

Ingredients:

- 4 salmon fillets
- 2 cups mixed vegetables (such as bell peppers, zucchini, cherry tomatoes, and onions), chopped
- 2 tablespoons olive oil
- 2 cloves garlic, minced
- 1 teaspoon dried herbs (such as thyme, rosemary, or oregano)
- Salt and pepper to taste
- Lemon wedges for serving

Instructions:

1. Preheat the oven to 400°F (200°C).
2. Place the salmon fillets on a baking sheet lined with parchment paper.

3. In a large bowl, toss the mixed vegetables with olive oil, minced garlic, dried herbs, salt, and pepper until evenly coated.

4. Spread the vegetables out in a single layer on another baking sheet lined with parchment paper.

5. Place both baking sheets in the oven and bake for 15-20 minutes, or until the salmon is cooked through and the vegetables are tender and lightly browned.

6. Remove the baking sheets from the oven and serve the salmon fillets with the roasted vegetables.

7. Squeeze fresh lemon juice over the top before serving.

Enjoy your baked salmon with roasted vegetables for a flavorful and satisfying dinner that's as delicious as it is nutritious.

(Note: Carb counting and nutritional information are approximate and may vary depending on specific ingredients and portion sizes used.)

Dinner Recipe 2: Turkey and Vegetable Stir-Fry

<u>Introduction:</u>

Delight your taste buds with a savory turkey and vegetable stir-fry, a diabetes-friendly dinner option that's bursting with flavor and packed with nutrients. With its combination of lean protein and colorful vegetables, this hearty meal will leave you feeling satisfied and nourished.

Carb Counting: Approximately 25 grams of carbohydrates per serving.

<u>Nutritional Information:</u>
- Calories: 300
- Total Fat: 12g
- Saturated Fat: 2g
- Cholesterol: 80mg
- Sodium: 450mg
- Total Carbohydrates: 25g
- Dietary Fiber: 7g
- Sugars: 8g
- Protein: 20g

Serving Size: 1 bowl

Prep Time: 20 minutes

<u>Ingredients:</u>

- 1 lb ground turkey
- 2 cups mixed vegetables (such as bell peppers, broccoli, snap peas, and carrots), chopped
- 2 cloves garlic, minced
- 1 tablespoon ginger, minced
- 2 tablespoons low-sodium soy sauce
- 1 tablespoon rice vinegar
- 1 teaspoon sesame oil
- Salt and pepper to taste
- Cooked brown rice or quinoa for serving

<u>Instructions:</u>

1. Heat a large skillet or wok over medium-high heat. Add the ground turkey and cook, breaking it apart with a spatula, until browned and cooked through.
2. Add the mixed vegetables, minced garlic, and minced ginger to the skillet and stir-fry for 3-4 minutes, or until the vegetables are crisp-tender.
3. In a small bowl, whisk together the soy sauce, rice vinegar, and sesame oil.
4. Pour the sauce over the turkey and vegetables in the skillet and stir to combine.

5. Cook for an additional 1-2 minutes, or until the sauce is heated through.

6. Season with salt and pepper to taste.

7. Serve the turkey and vegetable stir-fry over cooked brown rice or quinoa.

Enjoy your savory turkey and vegetable stir-fry for a delicious and nutritious dinner that's sure to satisfy your cravings.

(Note: Carb counting and nutritional information are approximate and may vary depending on specific ingredients and portion sizes used.)

Dinner Recipe 3: Lentil and Vegetable Soup

Introduction:
Warm your soul with a comforting bowl of lentil and vegetable soup, a diabetes-friendly dinner option that's hearty, healthy, and delicious. Packed with fiber-rich lentils and an assortment of colorful vegetables, this nourishing soup will leave you feeling satisfied and content.

Carb Counting: Approximately 30 grams of carbohydrates per serving.

Nutritional Information:

- Calories: 250
- Total Fat: 5g
- Saturated Fat: 1g
- Cholesterol: 0mg
- Sodium: 600mg
- Total Carbohydrates: 30g
- Dietary Fiber: 10g
- Sugars: 8g
- Protein: 15g

Serving Size: 1 bowl

Prep Time: 30 minutes

Ingredients:

- 1 cup dried green or brown lentils, rinsed and drained
- 4 cups low-sodium vegetable broth
- 2 cups mixed vegetables (such as carrots, celery, onions, and potatoes), diced
- 2 cloves garlic, minced

- 1 teaspoon dried herbs (such as thyme, rosemary, or oregano)
- Salt and pepper to taste
- Fresh parsley for garnish

Instructions:

1. In a large pot, combine the dried lentils, vegetable broth, mixed vegetables, minced garlic, and dried herbs.
2. Bring the soup to a boil over medium-high heat, then reduce the heat to low and simmer for 20-25 minutes, or until the lentils and vegetables are tender.
3. Season the soup with salt and pepper to taste.
4. Ladle the soup into bowls and garnish with fresh parsley before serving.

Enjoy your hearty lentil and vegetable soup for a cozy and comforting dinner that's perfect for chilly evenings.

(Note: Carb counting and nutritional information are approximate and may vary depending on specific ingredients and portion sizes used.)

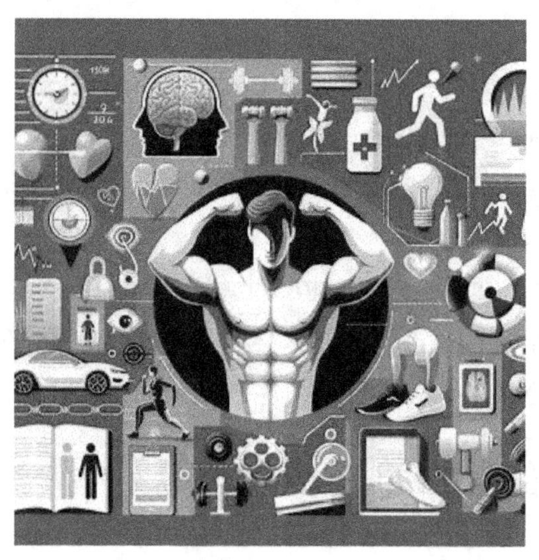

Physical Activity and Exercise Routines

Chapter 4: Physical Activity and Exercise Routines

A crucial component of controlling Type 2 diabetes is exercise. You can regulate your blood sugar levels more effectively, decrease weight, and lower your risk of heart disease and stroke by engaging in regular physical activity. Additionally, exercise can strengthen your bones and muscles, improve your circulation, and increase your mood and energy.

Consider the following exercise categories:

Exercises that are aerobic include jogging, swimming, biking, hiking, and walking.

• Resistance training: Strengthening and muscle-building exercises of this kind. Examples include lifting weights, utilizing resistance bands, or performing exercises like pushups and squats using only your body weight.

Exercises for flexibility and stretching can help you increase your range of motion and lessen stiffness. Pilates, yoga, and tai chi are a few examples.

• Balance drills: These drills help you become more coordinated and stable. Examples include doing heel lifts, walking heel to toe, and standing on one leg.

Regardless of the workout you select, it's crucial to see y hiour doctor before beginning a new fitness regimen. They can assist you in developing a plan that is suitable for your needs, safe, and effective. Additionally, it's crucial to hydrate well and warm up and cool down before and after each exercise session.

Regular exercise can significantly improve your health and assist you in controlling your diabetes. Therefore, if you're searching for a way to enhance your general health, think about including physical activity in your daily schedule.

Physical Activity and Exercise Routines and How They're Carried Out

1. Dance Fitness Class:

Immerse yourself in the rhythm and energy of a dance fitness class, where you can groove to the music while getting a full-body workout. Whether it's Zumba, hip-hop, or salsa, dancing not only burns calories but also improves cardiovascular health, coordination, and mood.

How it's carried out:

Attend a dance fitness class at your local gym or community center, or follow along with online dance workout videos in the comfort of your own home. Let the music guide you as you move your body to the beat, incorporating various dance steps and choreography to keep things fun and engaging.

2. Interval Training:

Get your heart pumping with interval training, a high-intensity workout that alternates between bursts of vigorous exercise and short periods of rest or lower-intensity activity. This type of workout is excellent for improving cardiovascular fitness, burning calories, and boosting metabolism.

How it's carried out:

Choose your preferred form of aerobic exercise, such as running, cycling, or jumping rope. Start with a brief warm-up, then alternate between short bursts of intense effort (e.g., sprinting or cycling at maximum intensity) and periods of recovery (e.g., walking or slow jogging) for a set amount of time or repetitions. Finish with a cooldown and stretching to prevent injury and promote flexibility.

3. Outdoor Circuit Training:

Take your workout outdoors and enjoy the fresh air with an outdoor circuit training routine. This versatile workout combines strength training exercises with cardiovascular intervals, using your body weight or portable equipment like resistance bands or suspension trainers.

How it's carried out:

Find a suitable outdoor location with space for various exercises, such as a park or playground. Design a circuit that includes a mix of exercises targeting different muscle groups, such as squats, lunges, push-ups, jumping jacks, and mountain climbers. Perform each exercise for a set amount of time or repetitions, then move on to the next exercise with minimal rest in between. Complete the circuit for multiple rounds, adjusting the intensity and difficulty as needed to challenge yourself.

4. Nature Walk or Hike:

Connect with nature while improving your health with a leisurely nature walk or a more challenging hike through scenic trails. Walking or hiking in natural environments not only provides physical benefits but also reduces stress, boosts mood, and promotes mental well-being.

How it's carried out:

Choose a trail or nature reserve suitable for your fitness level and preferences, whether it's a paved path through a local park or a rugged trail in the mountains. Dress appropriately for the weather and terrain, wear comfortable footwear, and bring water and snacks for hydration and energy. Start with a gentle warm-up and gradually increase your pace as you walk or hike, taking breaks as needed to rest and admire the surroundings. Pay attention to your surroundings and immerse yourself in the sights, sounds, and sensations of nature as you move your body and nourish your soul.

5. Swimming:

Dive into the refreshing waters of swimming for a full-body workout that's gentle on the joints and invigorating for the spirit. Whether you're doing laps in the pool or enjoying a leisurely swim, swimming improves cardiovascular health, builds muscle strength, and enhances flexibility.

How it's carried out:

Head to your local swimming pool or natural body of water and don your swimsuit and goggles. Start with a warm-up by swimming easy laps or treading water for a few minutes. Then, engage in various swimming strokes, such as freestyle, breaststroke, backstroke, and butterfly, for a well-rounded workout. Focus on maintaining proper form and breathing rhythm as you glide through the water, feeling the stress melt away with each stroke.

6. Indoor Cycling (Spin Class):

Pedal your way to fitness and euphoria with an indoor cycling class, also known as spin class. With energizing music, motivating instructors, and adjustable resistance levels, indoor cycling offers a high-intensity cardiovascular workout that strengthens the legs, boosts endurance, and uplifts the spirit.

How it's carried out:

Attend a spin class at your local gym or fitness studio, where you'll be guided through a series of simulated rides, hill climbs, sprints, and intervals on a stationary bike. Set your resistance level and follow the instructor's cues as you pedal to the rhythm of the music, pushing yourself to reach new levels of speed and intensity. Feel the adrenaline coursing through your veins as you conquer each hill and cross the finish line, empowered and exhilarated by the journey.

7. Kickboxing or Martial Arts:

Unleash your inner warrior with kickboxing or martial arts training, a dynamic and empowering way to improve physical fitness, mental focus, and self-confidence. Whether you're throwing punches, kicks, or grappling techniques, kickboxing and martial arts workouts challenge your body and mind while teaching valuable self-defense skills.

How it's carried out:

Join a kickboxing class or martial arts studio in your area, where you'll learn basic techniques and drills under the guidance of experienced instructors. Warm up with dynamic stretches and shadowboxing, then progress to partner drills, pad work, and bag work to refine your striking and defensive abilities. Embrace the discipline and camaraderie of the martial arts community as you push your limits, overcome obstacles, and emerge stronger and more resilient than ever before.

8. Dance Therapy or Movement Meditation:

Embark on a transformative journey of self-discovery and healing with dance therapy or movement meditation, modalities that integrate movement, music, and mindfulness to promote holistic well-being. Through expressive movement and guided meditation, dance therapy and movement meditation release tension, reduce stress, and cultivate inner peace and harmony.

How it's carried out:

Participate in a dance therapy workshop or movement meditation class led by certified practitioners or therapists trained in somatic practices. Begin by centering yourself through deep breathing and grounding exercises, then allow the music to guide your movements as you explore different rhythms, shapes, and emotions. Express yourself freely and authentically, releasing any tension or resistance held in the body and inviting in a sense of flow and connection with the present moment.

9. Group Fitness Classes (e.g., Bootcamp, HIIT, Barre):

Join forces with like-minded individuals and embark on a journey of fitness and camaraderie with group fitness classes, such as bootcamp, HIIT (high-intensity interval training), or barre. These dynamic and diverse workouts offer a mix of cardio, strength training, and flexibility exercises, tailored to challenge and inspire participants of all fitness levels.

How it's carried out:

Enroll in a group fitness class at your local gym, studio, or community center, where certified instructors will lead you through a series of exercises and routines designed to target different muscle groups and energy systems. Whether you're sweating it out in a bootcamp-style circuit, pushing your limits in a HIIT session, or toning and sculpting with barre exercises, feel the support and encouragement of your fellow classmates as you strive toward your fitness goals together. Celebrate your progress and achievements as you emerge stronger, fitter, and more empowered with each exhilarating workout.

10. Outdoor Adventure Activities (e.g., Hiking, Rock Climbing, Kayaking):

Embark on an outdoor adventure and reconnect with nature while engaging in exhilarating physical activities such as hiking, rock climbing, or kayaking. These outdoor pursuits not only provide an excellent workout for the body but also nourish the soul, fostering a sense of awe, gratitude, and connection with the natural world.

How it's carried out:

Choose your preferred outdoor adventure activity and find a suitable location, whether it's a scenic hiking trail, a towering rock face, or a tranquil river or lake. Equip yourself with appropriate gear and safety equipment, and embark on your outdoor journey with a sense of curiosity and adventure. Feel the exhilaration of conquering new heights, navigating challenging terrain, or gliding through the water, immersing yourself in the beauty and majesty of the great outdoors. Let the rhythm of nature guide your movements as you breathe in the fresh air, soak up the sunshine, and embrace the thrill of exploration and discovery.

Chapter 5 : Medications and Treatments

A chronic illness, type 2 diabetes can be controlled through dietary adjustments, medication, and other therapies. Maintaining blood glucose levels within a specific range is the main objective of treatment to lower the risk of problems.

An essential component of type 2 diabetes management is medication. It is used to lower the risk of problems and help keep blood glucose levels within the desired range. It is possible to utilize insulin, sulfonylureas, meglitinides, thiazolidinediones, dipeptidyl peptidase-4 inhibitors, and glucagon-like peptide-1 agonists among other types of medication. Every medicine has a unique mechanism of action and a unique set of potential adverse effects.

Changes in lifestyle are also crucial for managing type 2 diabetes. Stress reduction, a nutritious diet, and regular exercise can all help keep blood sugar levels within the desired range. It's crucial to stop smoking because it raises your chance of problems.

Type 2 diabetes can be managed with additional therapies. These include undergoing weight loss surgery, using an insulin pump, and continuously monitoring glucose levels.

To properly control type 2 diabetes, it may occasionally be required to use a mix of prescription drugs, lifestyle modifications, and other treatments. The ideal treatment strategy for your particular needs should be determined in collaboration with a healthcare professional.

Chapter 6: Living Well with Type 2 Diabetes

With the appropriate attitude and lifestyle, living well with Type 2 Diabetes is feasible. Chronic Type 2 Diabetes alters how your body metabolizes blood sugar, which results in elevated blood sugar levels. Although there is no cure for this condition, it can be managed with the right care.

The first step in delaying or preventing the onset of Type 2 Diabetes is to take preventive measures. This entails getting regular exercise, following a healthy diet, keeping a healthy weight, and limiting or abstaining from alcohol and tobacco use.

Second, it's crucial to periodically check your blood sugar levels. You can check your blood sugar levels at home using a glucose meter or by going to the doctor for routine blood sugar checks.

Thirdly, it's crucial to take your prescriptions exactly as your physician has instructed. This includes drugs that lower blood sugar levels and drugs that lessen your chance of developing disease-related problems.

Fourth, it's crucial to adopt a healthy lifestyle. This entails maintaining a regular exercise schedule and eating a balanced diet low in salt, sugar, and fat. Get proper rest and manage your stress as well.

For support and direction, it's crucial to keep in touch with your doctor and other medical experts. They can assist you in modifying your lifestyle to maintain healthy blood sugar levels.

With the correct attitude, a change in lifestyle, and support, living well with Type 2 Diabetes is feasible. You can control your diabetes and live a healthy, meaningful life with help and dedication.

Chapter 7: Nutrition and Meal Planning

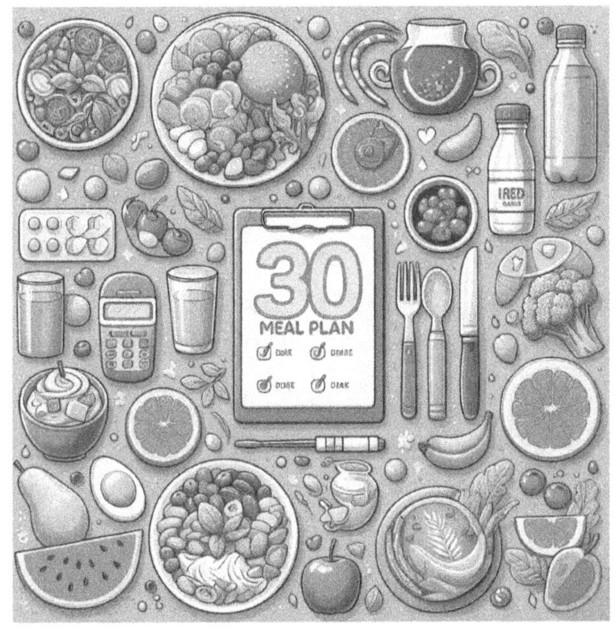

30 days meal plan and shopping list

<u>**Week 1:**</u>

Day 1:

- Breakfast: Oatmeal with almond milk and fresh fruit.
- Lunch: Salad with grilled chicken, mixed greens, tomatoes, cucumbers, and olive oil vinaigrette.
- Snack: Fruit and cottage cheese.
- Dinner: Roasted veggies and baked salmon.

Day 2:

- Breakfast: Whole-wheat bread with banana and peanut butter.
- Lunch: Baked sweet potato with salsa and black beans.
- Snack: Greek yogurt, chopped nuts, and dried fruit.
- Dinner: Grilled shrimp and stir-fried vegetables.

Day 3:

- Breakfast: Eggs scrambled with bell peppers and mushrooms.
- Lunch: Quinoa and black bean tortilla.
- Snack: Hummus-topped celery sticks.
- Dinner: Vegan chili.

Day 4:

- Breakfast: Greek yogurt and fruit smoothie.
- Lunch: Turkey sandwich with lettuce, tomato, and avocado.
- Snack: Apple slices with peanut butter.
- Dinner: Roasted chicken and broccoli.

Day 5:

- Breakfast: Chia-seed-infused overnight oats.
- Lunch: Tzatziki and baked falafel.
- Snack: Hummus and carrot sticks.
- Dinner: Lenten soup.

Day 6:

- Breakfast: Egg-white omelet with bell peppers and spinach.
- Lunch: Salad with grilled salmon, mixed greens, tomatoes, and balsamic vinaigrette.
- Snack: Almond butter on celery sticks.
- Dinner: Baked sweet potatoes with salsa and black beans.

Day 7:

- Breakfast: Avocado on whole wheat toast.
- Lunch: Quinoa and veggie stir-fry.

- Snack:Greek yogurt and granola.
- Dinner: Grilled shrimp and a green salad.

Week 2:

Day 8:

- Breakfast: Oatmeal with berries and almonds.
- Lunch: Tzatziki and baked falafel.
- Snack: Apple slices with peanut butter.
- Dinner: Eggplant Parmesan.

Day 9:

- Breakfast: Greek yogurt and fruit smoothie.
- Lunch: Salad with grilled chicken, mixed greens, tomatoes, and olive oil vinaigrette.
- Snack: Hummus and carrot sticks.
- Dinner: Lenten soup.

Day 10:

- Breakfast: Eggs scrambled with bell peppers and mushrooms.
- Lunch: Quinoa and black bean tortilla.
- Snack: Almond butter on celery sticks.
- Dinner: Roasted veggies and baked salmon.

Day 11:

- Breakfast: Whole-wheat bread with banana and peanut butter.
- Lunch: Salad with grilled salmon, mixed greens, tomatoes, and balsamic vinaigrette.
- Snack: Greek yogurt, chopped nuts, and dried fruit.
- Dinner: Vegan chili.

Day 12:

- Breakfast: Chia-seed-infused overnight oats.
- Lunch: Turkey sandwich with lettuce, tomato, and avocado.
- Snack: Fruit and cottage cheese.
- Dinner: Roasted chicken and broccoli.

Day 13:

- Breakfast: Egg-white omelet with bell peppers and spinach.
- Lunch: Baked sweet potato with salsa and black beans.
- Snack: Hummus-topped celery sticks.
- Dinner: Grilled shrimp and stir-fried vegetables.

Day 14:

- Breakfast: Oatmeal with almond milk and fresh fruit.
- Lunch: Quinoa and veggie stir-fry.
- Snack: Apple slices with peanut butter.
- Dinner: Eggplant Parmesan.

Week 3:

Day 15:

- Breakfast: Greek yogurt and fruit smoothie.
- Lunch: Salad with grilled chicken, mixed greens, tomatoes, and olive oil vinaigrette.
- Snack: Hummus and carrot sticks.
- Dinner: Lenten soup.

Day 16:

- Breakfast: Avocado on whole wheat toast.
- Lunch: Tzatziki and baked falafel.
- Snack: Almond butter on celery sticks.
- Dinner: Roasted veggies and baked salmon.

Day 17:

- Breakfast: Eggs scrambled with bell peppers and mushrooms.
- Lunch: Quinoa and black bean tortilla.

- Snack: Greek yogurt and granola.
- Dinner: Vegan chili.

Day 18:

- Breakfast: Chia-seed-infused overnight oats.
- Lunch: Salad with grilled salmon, mixed greens, tomatoes, and balsamic vinaigrette.
- Snack: Fruit and cottage cheese.
- Dinner: Roasted chicken and broccoli.

Day 19:

- Breakfast: Whole-wheat bread with banana and peanut butter.
- Lunch: Baked sweet potato with salsa and black beans.
- Snack: Apple slices with peanut butter.
- Dinner: Grilled shrimp and a green salad.

Day 20:

- Breakfast: Egg-white omelet with bell peppers and spinach.
- Lunch: Salad with grilled chicken, mixed greens, tomatoes, cucumbers, and olive oil vinaigrette.
- Snack: Hummus-topped celery sticks.
- Dinner: Lenten soup.

<u>**Week 4:**</u>

Day 21:

- Breakfast: Oatmeal with berries and almonds.
- Lunch: Tzatziki and baked falafel.
- Snack: Hummus and carrot sticks.
- Dinner: Egg plant Parmesan.

Day 22:

- Breakfast: Greek yogurt and fruit smoothie.
- Lunch: Salad with grilled salmon, mixed greens, tomatoes, and balsamic vinaigrette.
- Snack: Greek yogurt, chopped nuts, and dried fruit.
- Dinner: Roasted veggies and baked salmon.

Day 23:

- Breakfast: Avocado on whole wheat toast.
- Lunch: Quinoa and veggie stir-fry.
- Snack: Hummus and carrot sticks.
- Dinner: Vegan chili.

Day 24:

- Breakfast: Eggs scrambled with bell peppers and mushrooms.

- Lunch: Baked sweet potato with salsa and black beans.
- Snack: Almond butter on celery sticks.
- Dinner: Grilled shrimp and stir-fried vegetables.

Day 25:

- Breakfast: Oatmeal with almond milk and fresh fruit.
- Lunch: Quinoa and black bean tortilla.
- Snack: Fruit and cottage cheese.
- Dinner: Lenten soup.

Day 26:

- Breakfast: Whole-wheat bread with banana and peanut butter.
- Lunch: Salad with grilled chicken, mixed greens, tomatoes, cucumbers, and olive oil vinaigrette.
- Snack: Hummus and carrot sticks.
- Dinner: Roasted veggies and baked salmon.

Day 27:

- Breakfast: Greek yogurt and fruit smoothie.
- Lunch: Tzatziki and baked falafel.
- Snack: Apple slices with peanut butter.
- Dinner: Eggplant Parmesan.

Day 28:

- Breakfast: Egg-white omelet with bell peppers and spinach.
- Lunch: Salad with grilled salmon, mixed greens, tomatoes, and balsamic vinaigrette.
- Snack: Almond butter on celery sticks.
- Dinner: Grilled shrimp and a green salad.

Day 29:

- Breakfast: Oatmeal with berries and almonds.
- Lunch: Quinoa and veggie stir-fry.
- Snack: Hummus-topped celery sticks.
- Dinner: Lenten soup.

Day 30:

- Breakfast: Avocado on whole wheat toast.
- Lunch: Salad with grilled chicken, mixed greens, tomatoes, and olive oil vinaigrette.
- Snack: Greek yogurt and granola.
- Dinner: Roasted veggies and baked salmon.

Shopping List:

- - Oatmeal
- - Almond milk

- - Fresh fruit (e.g., berries, bananas, apples)
- - Mixed greens
- - Chicken breast
- - Tomatoes
- - Cucumbers
- - Olive oil
- - Vinaigrette
- - Cottage cheese
- - Whole-wheat bread
- - Peanut butter
- - Sweet potatoes
- - Salsa
- - Black beans
- - Greek yogurt
- - Nuts (e.g., almonds, peanuts)
- - Dried fruit
- - Salmon
- - Eggs
- - Bell peppers
- - Mushrooms
- - Quinoa
- - Tortillas
- - Hummus
- - Celery
- - Shrimp

- - Stir-fry vegetables
- - Avocado
- - Tzatziki
- - Falafel
- - Lenten soup ingredients (e.g., lentils, vegetables)
- - Eggplant
- - Lettuce
- - Turkey
- - Granola

Conclusion

In conclusion, managing type 2 diabetes is not just about following a strict diet or exercise regimen; it's about embracing a holistic approach to health and well-being. Throughout this book, we've explored the various aspects of living with type 2 diabetes, from understanding the condition and its risk factors to implementing proactive strategies for better management.

We've delved into the importance of nutrition and provided a plethora of delicious and nutritious meal ideas, ensuring that eating well is not only beneficial for controlling blood sugar levels but also enjoyable and satisfying. From hearty breakfasts to flavorful dinners, each meal has been crafted with care to nourish both the body and the soul.

We've also emphasized the significance of physical activity in diabetes management, showcasing a diverse range of exercises and activities that promote cardiovascular health, strength, flexibility, and overall well-being. Whether it's swimming laps in the pool, cycling through scenic trails, or practicing yoga in the comfort of your home, there's a form of exercise for everyone to enjoy.

Furthermore, we've discussed the importance of regular monitoring, medication adherence, stress management, and foot care in maintaining optimal health with type 2 diabetes. By staying proactive and vigilant, individuals can minimize the risk of complications and enjoy a fulfilling and vibrant life despite their diagnosis.

But perhaps most importantly, this book has emphasized the power of resilience, determination, and community support in the journey with type 2 diabetes. Living with a chronic condition can be challenging, but with the right tools, knowledge, and mindset, individuals can overcome obstacles and thrive.

As we conclude this journey together, let us remember that managing type 2 diabetes is not just about managing numbers on a screen or adhering to a strict regimen; it's about embracing life with courage, compassion, and optimism. Together, we can empower each other to live our best lives and redefine what it means to thrive with type 2 diabetes.